The
Ultimate
Diet
Counter

The
Ultimate
Diet
Counter

by

Charles and Maureen Clark

Vermilion

First published in the United Kingdom in 2003 by
Vermilion, an imprint of Ebury Press
Random House UK Ltd.
Random House
20 Vauxhall Bridge Road
London SW1V 2SA

Random House Australia (Pty) Limited
20 Alfred Street, Milsons Point, Sydney,
New South Wales 2061, Australia

Random House New Zealand Limited
18 Poland Road, Glenfield,
Auckland 10, New Zealand

Random House (Pty) Limited
Endulini, 5A Jubilee Road, Parktown 2193, South Africa

Random House UK Limited Reg. No. 954009
www.randomhouse.co.uk
Papers used by Vermilion are natural, recyclable products
made from wood grown in sustainable forests.

A CIP catalogue record is available for this book from the
British Library.

ISBN: 0091889715

The advice offered in this book is not intended to be a substitute for the advice
and counsel of your personal physician. Always consult a medical practitioner
before embarking on a diet, or a course of exercise. Neither the author nor the
publisher can be held responsible for any loss or claim arising out of the use, or
misuse, of the suggestions made, or the failure to take medical advice.

Printed and bound in Great Britain by
Bookmarque Ltd, Croydon, Surrey

Contents

Acknowledgements

We thank our children, David and Heather, for their unbiased critiques on the many recipes they have tested for us. Their criticism was always constructive, if perhaps not always appreciated at the time.

And, of course, the wonderful team at Vermilion for their consistent support and advice.

Introduction

Dieting is easy! There are only two rules you need to know to lose weight easily – and we don't mean starving yourself, which is the basis of calorie-controlled diets:

1   Reduce carbohydrates
2   Eat a healthy, balanced diet.

You will see that these simple rules don't mention reducing calories, or eating less. On the contrary, there is no need to eat less on an effective, medically-based weight-loss diet. You should *never* be hungry on a diet, and you will certainly never be hungry on this diet. You can programme your body to burn body fat by reducing your carbohydrate intake to low levels. Remember, you need proteins, fats, vitamins and minerals for health, *but you don't need refined carbohydrates*. Refined carbohydrates have virtually no nutritional value whatsoever, they just provide energy, which we can easily obtain from essential proteins and fats. And the excess energy from excess carbohydrates in the diet is deposited as body fat. Carbohydrates in your diet are actually the factor controlling the deposition of body fat; if you reduce carbohydrates in your diet, you will automatically start losing the body fat you have been desperately trying to lose.

This book provides the carbohydrate values of individual food groups, which enables you to lose weight according to the method described in *The New High Protein Diet* (published by

Vermilion). The aim of this book is to give you *simple guidelines for quick and effective weight loss, without hunger.* Follow the simple guidelines in *The New High Protein Diet* and you are guaranteed to lose weight quickly, easily – without hunger cravings and without pain.

Effective dieting to lose *fat* not just *weight* (which includes our all-important body protein) requires the restriction of carbohydrates – not calories or fats as you may have been previously advised. But to achieve this goal you need to know the approximate carbohydrate content of the foods commonly included in our diet (even the 'bad' ones, so that you can avoid them!). This needs to be as simple as possible, hence the need for a small pocket diet book. It is not the intention of this book to attempt to provide all of the carbohydrate values for all foods. Apart from being impossible, this would also defeat the aim of the book, which is *to make effective dieting as simple as possible.* The aim is to provide you with a simple and effective system of dieting, by indicating food groups which are unrestricted, and those which are excluded. So you don't have to count carbohydrates or calories, but merely enjoy virtually unlimited foods from the appropriate categories. It is that simple!

And it must be emphasized that these values are *approximate values only.* It is intended as a guide for dieting, not an exact scientific measurement – because despite the information given in some texts on this subject, it is not possible to give an *exact* carbohydrate measurement for all foods. Why? Well the simple answer is that foods vary. For example, apples are all different sizes, meats contain different proportions of fat per unit weight, and the same type of biscuit from different manufacturers has different proportions of carbohydrates and fats (although not much protein, for obvious reasons). So it's meaningless to give you seemingly exact proportions of carbohydrates for each type of food when the nature of the measurement is, by definition, variable.

In summary, food is a variable commodity so the values given in this booklet are approximations only – but probably the most accurate approximations you will ever need to ensure an effective low-carbohydrate diet.

The other reason that the values in the book are only approximations is that the aim of this diet is *that you don't have to count – calories or carbohydrates!* So you won't find all foods in this book, but you will find *all food groups*. This diet is a lifestyle, not just a way of losing weight. It is not natural, or necessary, to constantly check the calorie content of foods to diet effectively and healthily. In this system, instead of diligently checking all foods for their carbohydrate content, you merely have to learn the *principles* of the diet – which food groups are included without restriction (like meat and fish), and which groups are completely excluded (like rice and pasta) – and you will lose weight the easy and certain way. If you adhere to the foods which are low in carbohydrates – which are clearly marked in each list with an asterisk (*) – *you won't have to count anything.*

You only have to count carbohydrates if you decide to add foods which have a high carbohydrate content into the diet *occasionally,* such as a chocolate biscuit. But it's much easier to simply adhere to the unrestricted foods – of which there are many – and then you don't have any counting to do. After all, it would be pointless to design a diet which merely replaces counting calories by counting carbohydrates. This diet is specifically designed to be much simpler – and certainly more effective – than the old calorie diet: on this diet you can eat *almost as much as you like* of the unrestricted foods, and still lose fat!

The essential rule of the diet is that you must restrict carbo-hydrates to *40–60 grams per day*, and the best way to be sure of keeping within the 40–60 grams of carbohydrate per day limit is to acquire the habit of reading the labels on packaged foods. This will give you a quick and simple answer to the carbo-hydrate content, but if you're not sure of the carbohydrate content, *leave it on the shelf.*

The rationale behind the success of a low-carbohydrate diet (and the failure of other diets, especially low-fat diets) is explained in detail in *The New High Protein Diet*, but for sim-plicity it is worth repeating the Golden Rules of the diet; follow these, and you will definitely lose fat quickly and easily.

Restricted Foods

- Carbohydrates *must* be severely restricted to low levels
- Restrict fruit
- Alcohol: no beer, cider or fortified/sweet wines (sherry, port, Madeira)
- Avoid coffee, if possible; if not, have decaffeinated coffee
- Virtually no milk – even skimmed milk
- No fruit juices
- No pulses or grains in the early stage of the diet
- No carbonated soft drinks, except the 'diet' variety

Foods included in diet

- Virtually no restriction on the amount of protein
- Virtually no restriction on 'pure' fats
- Include eggs in your diet (up to 2 per day)
- Include fresh vegetables

- Alcohol: dry wine (white or red) and spirits, in moderation
- Drink tea
- 'Diet' soft drinks only

General advice

- Stir-fry food as much as possible
- Incorporate garlic and ginger in your diet
- Eat a substantial breakfast
- Eat an orange (or take a vitamin C supplement) every day
- Include herbs and spices to your diet
- Multivitamin supplements – 1 per day
- Regular exercise
- Measure shape before weight
- Vary your menu as much as possible

The book is divided into 22 sections, with general food headings (for example 'Biscuits, Cakes and Pastries') which provide quick and easy reference to assist your effective dieting. The beginning of each section tells you whether this food group is good for the diet or not! The advice is based on the Golden Rules, but removes all the hard work. You simply look up the section, and it tells you in straightforward terms whether you should include this particular food in the diet.

Finally, there is a section on the nutritional value of food. This explains in simple terms the nutrition we obtain from food, what we require, and, perhaps more importantly, the myths about nutrition that are simply not correct.

This book provides the *only* 4 essential items of relevant information you need for successful, healthy dieting: carbohydrate content, calories, protein content and nutritional value.

Carbohydrate content is essential for successful weight loss; protein content and nutritional value are essential for health; and calories are for interest only, *as you do not need to count calories on this diet.*

1 Carbohydrate content

The only important factor for successful weight loss is carbohydrate content. You must keep your carbohydrate intake *below 60 grams per day* (and preferably below 40 grams per day) for the diet to be effective. Too much carbohydrate, and the diet will inevitably fail.

2 Calories

Each section will give the energy content (in calories) *for interest only.* This is of no relevance to the diet whatsoever, but is merely included to prove to you that you can consume foods of high calorific content and still lose weight easily.

3 Protein Content

Proteins are essential for health. Amino acids from proteins are the 'building blocks' of life, without which we cannot survive, so the protein content of foods is of paramount importance to our continued health. The book gives a simple symbolic measure in incremental stages (from + to + + + +) of the protein content of various foods to provide you with a straightforward guide to their real protein value, which is all you need in order to select foods appropriately. Complex statistics of protein content are confusing and of little practical value.

4 Nutritional value

The measure of nutritional value of individual foods takes into account all of the potentially healthy properties of the food, with particular emphasis on essential nutritional content (from amino acids, essential fats, vitamins and minerals) and antioxidant properties. Once again, this complex medical equation has been condensed to a simple scoring system (from + to + + + +) so that you can instantly appreciate whether a particular food has any *real* nutritional value.

All of the foods recommended for inclusion in the diet have a high nutritional content – and they taste good! In general, foods with a high nutritional content are included with little or no restriction, so you can appreciate that this is a very healthy diet indeed.

There are three major groups of healthy foods, which have a high nutritional value, but which have to be excluded from the diet because of their high carbohydrate content: pulses, fruit and milk. The nutrients (vitamins, minerals and antioxidants) present in these foods are also present in many other foods which are included in the diet, without restriction, so there is no problem with deficiency by their exclusion. Of course, when you have reached your desired weight, you can bring these nutritious foods back into your diet, in moderation, in the weight-maintenance phase of the diet.

To make adherence to the diet as easily as possible, *an asterisk (*) is shown before all foods included without restriction in the diet*. Avoid the foods without an asterisk (or include them in the diet with extreme caution). This book has deliberately included the 'bad' foods (which you *must* avoid for effective dieting) so that you can see for yourself their high carbohydrate content.

All foods can be classified under the following categories, for simple reference:

Biscuits, Cakes and Pastries
Bread, Flour, Grains and Cereals
Chips, Crisps and Dips
Confectionery
Dairy Products
Desserts
Drinks
Eggs
Fast Food
Fish and Shellfish
Fruit
Herbs and Spices
Meat
Nuts
Oils, Mayonnaise and Dressings
Pasta and Noodles
Poultry
Pulses
Rice
Sauces, Mustards and Stock
Soups
Vegetables and Vegetable Products

In general, the following is a simple guide to foods *included* or *excluded* from the diet:

Foods included virtually without restriction

Fish and Shellfish
Herbs and Spices
Meat and Poultry
Oils and Dressings
Vegetables (except those with a high-carbohydrate content,
such as potatoes and parsnips)

Foods for which some restrictions apply

Dairy Products
Drinks
Eggs (up to 2 per day)
Fruit
Nuts
Sauces, Mustards and Stock
Soups

Foods excluded during the weight-loss phase

Biscuits, Cakes and Pastries
Bread, Flour, Grains and Cereals
Desserts and Sugars
Fast Food
Pasta and Noodles
Rice
Snack Foods

Keep within the *unrestricted* and *partially-restricted* categories, and you will lose weight easily and nutritiously.

Once again, *read the labels on packaged foods to determine their carbohydrate content,* and if you're uncertain about this, *leave the food on the shelf.*

Biscuits, Cakes and Pastries

Definitely excluded!

Biscuits, cakes and pastries vary tremendously in their carbohydrate content, depending on the manufacturer, but in general they consist of carbohydrates and fats – the worst possible combination for the dieter. They have very little nutritional value. All quantities are *per 100 grams*, with individual biscuit, slice of cake or pastry quoted in brackets below. Biscuits, cakes and pastries vary tremendously in size, shape and content, depending on the individual manufacturer, so the figures quoted are approximations only – even more so than in other categories.

Food Item	Carbohydrate (g)	Calories	Protein content	Nutritional value
Sweet biscuits				
Bourbon	70	500	+	+
(per biscuit)	8	60	+	+
Chocolate chip	70	500	+	+
(per biscuit)	7	50	+	+
Chocolate-coated	70	520	+	+
(per biscuit)	16	130	+	+
Cream	70	450	+	+
(per biscuit)	7	45	+	+
Crunch cream	64	520	+	+
(per biscuit)	9	75	+	+
Custard cream	65	500	+	+
(per biscuit)	8	65	+	+

Food Item	Carbohydrate (g)	Calories	Protein content	Nutritional value
DIGESTIVE				
chocolate	70	500	+	+
(per biscuit)	10	75	+	+
plain	65	450	+	+
(per biscuit)	10	70	+	+
Flapjack	57	475	+	+
(per biscuit)	13	110	+	+
Fruit-style	50	220	+	++
(per biscuit)	8	35	+	++
Ginger	80	450	+	+
(per biscuit)	8	45	+	+
Jaffa cake	70	370	+	+
(per biscuit)	10	20	+	+
Kit Kat	60	506	+	+
(per biscuit)	12	106	+	+
Kit Kat Orange	60	506	+	+
(per biscuit)	12	106	+	+
Rich tea style	75	460	+	+
(per biscuit)	6	35	+	+
SHORTBREAD				
round	65	500	+	+
(per slice)	10	80	+	+
Scotch finger	70	510	+	+
(per piece)	11	90	+	+
Shortcake	60	500	+	+
(per biscuit)	6	90	+	+
Wagon Wheel	68	425	+	+
(per biscuit)	27	170	+	+

Food Item	Carbohydrate (g)	Calories	Protein content	Nutritional value
Crackers & Crispbreads				
Cream cracker	65	450	+	+
(per cracker)	5	30	+	+
Oatcakes	65	450	+	+
(per biscuit)	6	45	+	+
Rye crispbread	70	330	+	+
(per crispbread)	6	25	+	+
Water biscuit	80	450	+	+
(per biscuit)	5	30	+	+
Wholemeal cracker	75	420	+	+
(per cracker)	5	30	+	+
Cakes				
Banana	70	420	+	+
(per slice: 50g)	35	210	+	+
Battenberg	50	380	+	+
(per slice: 50g)	25	190	+	+
Black Forest gateau	50	340	+	+
(per slice: 50g)	25	170	+	+
Carrot	45	400	+	+
(per slice: 50g)	23	200	+	+
Carrot and orange	55	440	+	+
(per cake: 30g)	15	122	+	+
Cheesecake	30	310	+	+
(per slice: 50g)	15	155	+	+
Chelsea bun	55	350	+	+
(per bun: 75g)	40	280	+	+
Cherry	60	400	+	+
(per slice: 50g)	30	200	+	+
Chocolate	60	400	+	+
(per slice: 50g)	30	200	+	+

Food Item	Carbohydrate (g)	Calories	Protein content	Nutritional value
Chocolate éclair	35	380	+	+
(per éclair)	25	270	+	+
Christmas	60	320	+	+
(per slice: 50g)	30	160	+	+
Cream bun	25	425	+	+
(per bun: 50g)	13	210	+	+
Crumpet	40	200	+	+
(per crumpet)	15	80	+	+
Doughnut				
cream	30	350	+	+
iced	45	420	+	+
sugar	50	340	+	+
Fruit	50	320	+	++
(per slice: 50g)	25	160	+	++
Fudge	50	400	+	+
(per slice: 50g)	25	200	+	+
Gateau	45	350	+	+
(per slice: 50g)	23	175	+	+
Hot cross bun	60	300	+	+
(per bun: 50g)	30	150	+	+
Iced fruit bun	45	300	+	+
(per bun: 75g)	33	225	+	+
Jam tart	63	390	+	+
(per tart: 33g)	21	130	+	+
Lemon curd tart	63	390	+	+
(per tart: 33g)	21	130	+	+
Lemon tart	33	415	+	+
(per slice: 50g)	17	208	+	+
Madeira	60	400	+	+
(per slice: 50g)	30	200	+	+

Food Item	Carbohydrate (g)	Calories	Protein content	Nutritional value
Manor House	49	400	+	+
(per slice: 50g)	25	200	+	+
Marble	60	400	+	+
(per slice: 50g)	30	200	+	+
Mini Jaffa cakes	73	398	+	+
(per cake)	5	26	+	+
Mud	60	420	+	+
(per slice: 50g)	30	210	+	+
SPONGE				
without jam	50	450	+	+
(per slice: 50g)	25	225	+	+
with jam	60	350	+	+
(per slice: 50g)	30	175	+	+
Strawberry sundae	53	385	+	+
(per cake: 45g)	24	175	+	+
Swiss roll	65	350	+	+
(per slice: 50g)	33	175	+	+
Viennese cakes	60	500	+	+
(per cake: 50g)	30	250	+	+
Whisky fruit loaf	59	260	+	+
(per slice: 50g)	30	130	+	+
Pastries (per 100g)				
Croissant	40	350	+	+
(per croissant)	25	210	+	+
DANISH				
apple	45	300	+	+
apricot	40	300	+	+
blueberry	40	300	+	+
chocolate	25	300	+	+
custard	35	300	+	+

Food Item	Carbohydrate (g)	Calories	Protein content	Nutritional value
Jams and Marmalades (per 100g)				
Jam, fruit	**69**	260	+	+
Jam, low sugar	**32**	123	+	+
Marmalade	**69**	260	+	+

Bread, Flour, Grains and Cereals

Definitely excluded!

Flour and cereals are virtually pure carbohydrate, so although there are slight differences between the carbohydrate content of various flours (and various manufacturers), all flour is basically excluded. Of course, a tablespoon of flour in a sauce, for example, to be divided between two people is a relatively negligible amount of carbohydrate per person, but larger amounts are definitely out.

Bread is essentially flour-based, and therefore very high in carbohydrates. Apart from wholemeal bread, which certainly has high nutritional qualities, most varieties of bread have very little intrinsic nutritional value, the only value emanating from the additives.

Read the labels for breads and pittas/tortillas. A single slice of bread can vary from 11 to 20 grams of carbohydrate (and often the bread marketed for 'slimmers' is actually higher in carbohydrate content per unit weight). So you have to read the labels, especially with breads. In the table below, the figures for carbohydrate content of bread is *per slice, or per roll, or per pitta or tortilla*, as this has more practical relevance than per 100 grams; because of the immense variability of sizes and shapes of bread loaves, the figures are approximate only.

Food Item	Carbohydrate (g)	Calories	Protein content	Nutritional value
Bread				
Bap	**30–41**	175–246	+/++	+/++
Bagel	**30**	140	+	+
Baguette	**23**	130	+	+
Bran loaf	**35**	130	+	+
Brown bread	**11–20**	53–97	+	+
Croissant	**22**	207	+	+
Date loaf	**25**	150	+	+
Focaccia	**30**	140	+	+
Fruit bread	**15**	77	+	+
Hamburger roll	**40**	215	+	+
Naan	**50**	340	+	+
Pitta	**12–50**	55–230	+	+
Roll	**25–33**	150–270	+	+
Tortilla	**12–25**	67–144	+	+
White bread	**11–20**	50–110	+	+
Wholemeal bread	**15-20**	77-102	+	++
Flour (per 100g)				
Arrowroot	**90**	350	+	+
Barley	**75**	350	+	+
Buckwheat	**75**	360	+	+
Corn	**90**	350	+	+
Maize	**75**	360	+	+
Rice	**80**	360	+	+
SOYA				
(full fat)	**23**	450	+++	+++
(low fat)	**28**	350	+++	+++
WHEAT				
plain/white	**77**	340	+	+
self-raising/white	**76**	330	+	+
wholemeal	**65**	320	+	++

Food Item	Carbohydrate (g)	Calories	Protein content	Nutritional value
Pastry (per 100g)				
Choux	**30**	350	+	+
Puff	**35**	400	+	+
Shortcrust	**55**	520	+	+
Wholemeal	**45**	500	+	+
Grains (per 100g)				
BARLEY				
pearl	**84**	360	+	+
wholegrain	**65**	300	+	++
Bulgar	**70**	330	+	+
Couscous	**72**	355	++	+
Oatmeal	**70**	400	+	+
Wheat germ	**45**	300	++	+++
Cereals (per 100g)				
Bran (natural)	**60**	270	+	++
Bran flakes	**70**	320	+	++
Chocolate rice pops	**95**	380	+	++
Coco Pops	**85**	380	+	++
Cornflakes	**85**	360	+	++
Corn Pops	**85**	380	+	++
Crisped rice	**90**	370	+	++
Fibre and fruit flakes	**75**	350	+	++
Fruit and nut flakes	**70**	350	+	++
Honey Loops	**77**	370	+	++
Honey Puffs	**90**	390	+	++
Honey Nut Cheerios	**78**	372	+	++
Muesli	**70**	360	+	++
Oats, instant	**70**	370	+	++
Porridge oats	**73**	400	+	++
Sugar-coated Cornflakes	**90**	370	+	++

Food Item	Carbohydrate (g)	Calories	Protein content	Nutritional value
Sugar puffed wheat	85	350	+	++
Sultana bran flakes	20	300	+	++

Chips, Crisps and Dips

Definitely excluded!

In general, snack foods have a high-carbohydrate content, but obviously you can substitute nuts for the standard snack foods. Nuts also have a high nutritional content (but try to avoid cashew nuts and sweet chestnuts, as they have a high carbohydrate content). The following are examples only; in general, all chips, crisps and dips are excluded from a low-carbohydrate diet.

Food Item	Carbohydrate (g)	Calories	Protein content	Nutritional value
Bombay mix (100g)	34	544	+++	++
Dipping chips (100g)	63	490	++	+
Dips (100g)				
Chilli cheese	9	550	+	+
Garlic and herb	7	370	+	+
Hot salsa	9	40	+	++
Popcorn	71	468	++	++
Potato crisps				
Cheese and onion (100g)	48	535	+	+
(per bag)	12	134	+	+
Potato hoops, curry flavour (100g)	55	525	+	+
(per bag)	28	260	+	+
Potato sticks (100g)	52	530	+	+
(per bag)	39	400	+	+

Food Item	Carbohydrate (g)	Calories	Protein content	Nutritional value
Prawn cocktail (100g)	49	535	+	+
(per bag)	12	134	+	+
Prawn crackers (100g)	60	534	+	+
Pringles Original (100g)	47	547	+	+
Ready salted (100g)	48	544	+	+
(per bag)	12	136	+	+
Roast beef (100g)	47	540	+	+
(per bag)	12	136	+	+
Roast chicken (100g)	46	550	+	+
(per bag)	12	140	+	+
Salt (100g)	45	570	+	+
(per bag)	12	140	+	+
Salt and vinegar (100g)	45	550	+	+
(per bag)	11	140	+	+
Sour cream and onion (100g)	65	435	+	+
(per bag)	14	94	+	+
Tomato (100g)	45	550	+	+
(per bag)	12	140	+	+

Confectionery

Definitely excluded!

Most confectionery and crisps are high in carbohydrate (with the exception of sugar-free chewing gum) and – even worse from the health point of view – also high in trans fats, which are definitely not healthy. All statistics relate to 100 grams of the product, to enable comparisons with other foods.

Remember, pure sugars are 100 per cent sugar! All forms of sugar – of every type and variety – are excluded, with the possible exception of very small quantities (less than 1 teaspoon) in cooking.

It is virtually impossible to lose weight unless you exclude all confectionery from your diet, but after you have lost weight you can reintroduce confectionery in moderation.

Food Item	Carbohydrate (g)	Calories	Protein content	Nutritional value
Chocolate				
Bounty	**56**	485	+	+
Cappuccino	**47**	530	+	+
Caramel whip	**52**	435	+	+
Chocolate, toffee and pecan bar	**58**	500	+	+
Chocolate whip	**58**	460	+	+
Coconut	**55**	500	+	+
Cooking	**60**	500	+	+
Double Decker	**65**	460	+	+
Flake	**55**	530	+	+
Fruit and nut	**55**	550	+	+

Food Item	Carbohydrate (g)	Calories	Protein content	Nutritional value
Fudge	72	445	+	+
Maltesers	61	490	++	+
Mars Bar	70	450	+	+
Milk	60	520	+	+
Milky Way	72	454	+	+
Mini eggs	68	495	+	+
(per egg)	2	15	+	+
Chocolate and nut bar	53	500	++	++
Orange	57	530	+	+
Ripple	59	528	+	+
Yorkie bar	58	526	+	+
Sweets				
Fudge	80	450	+	+
Liquorice	65	280	+	+
Strawberry sherbet sweets	93	380	+	+
CHEWING GUM				
*sugar-free	<1	40	tr	+
(per piece)	<1	4	tr	+
normal – with sugar	30	100	tr	+
(per piece)	3	10	tr	+
Sugar				
Caster	100	400	0	0
Demerara	100	394	0	0
Granulated	100	400	0	0
Icing	100	398	0	0

Dairy Products

Included without restriction!

Apart from yoghurt and milk, which should be restricted to less than 100 ml per day (enough for at least·10 cups of tea or coffee).

Foods included

Food Item	Carbohydrate (g)	Calories	Protein content	Nutritional value
*Butter and margarine (15g)				
*Standard	**0**	150	0	+
*Ghee (clarified)	**0**	150	0	+
*Margarine	**<1**	110	0	+
*Cheese (25g)				
*Bocconcini	**<1**	112	+++	+++
*Brie	**<1**	91	+++	+++
*Caerphilly	**<1**	94	+++	+++
*Camembert	**<1**	77	+++	+++
*Cheddar	**<1**	100	+++	+++
*Cheshire	**<1**	95	+++	+++
*Cottage	**<1**	25	+++	+++
*Cream cheese	**<1**	84	+++	+++
*Dubliner	**<1**	98	+++	+++
*Edam	**<1**	88	+++	+++
*Emmental	**<1**	95	+++	+++
*Feta	**<1**	70	+++	+++
*Gloucester	**<1**	100	+++	+++
*Goat's cheese	**<1**	50	+++	+++

Food Item	Carbohydrate (g)	Calories	Protein content	Nutritional value
*Gouda	<1	95	+++	+++
*Halloumi	<1	60	+++	+++
*Isle of Arran	<1	102	+++	+++
*Isle of Bute	<1	102	+++	+++
*Jarlsberg	<1	95	+++	+++
*Lancashire	<1	90	+++	+++
*Leicester	<1	100	+++	+++
*Mozzarella	<1	75	+++	+++
*Mull of Kintyre	<1	102	+++	+++
*Orkney	<1	102	+++	+++
*Parmesan	<1	110	+++	+++
*Philadelphia cream cheese	2	70	++	++
*Ricotta	<1	40	+++	+++
*Stilton	<1	92	+++	+++
*Wensleydale	<1	92	+++	+++
*Prepared cheeses (25g)				
*Cheese strings	<1	82	++++	++++
*(per stick: 21g)	<1	69	++++	++++
*Cheese strips	<1	86	+++	+++
*(per stick: 21g)	<1	73	+++	+++
*Cream (100ml)				
*Crème fraîche	3	380	+	++
*Double cream	3	460	++	++
*Single cream	3	330	++	++
*Soured cream	4	200	++	++

Foods excluded
(or included in very small quantities)

Food Item	Carbohydrate (g)	Calories	Protein content	Nutritional value
Milk (100ml)				
Cow's				
chocolate	**10**	82	++	++
condensed	**56**	330	++	++
evaporated	**11**	160	++	++
full-cream	**5**	66	++	+++
high-calcium	**5**	49	++	+++
semi-skimmed	**5**	50	++	+++
skimmed	**5**	35	++	+++
strawberry	**10**	81	++	++
UHT longlife	**5**	68	++	++
Goat's Milk	**4**	60	++	++
Soya	**1**	32	+	++
Yoghurt (100ml)				
Acidophilus	**8**	25	++	++
Blackcurrant	**17**	141	+	+
Blackberry and raspberry	**15**	125	+	+
Gooseberry with cream	**20**	190	+	+
Lemon curd	**20**	150	+	+
Raspberry and blackberry				
Creamy bio yoghurt	**11**	130	++	+
Rhubarb and cranberry	**17**	100	+	+
Strawberry bio yoghurt	**9**	114	+	+
Vanilla flavour with				
chocolate rice	**19**	120	+	++

Food Item	Carbohydrate (g)	Calories	Protein content	Nutritional value
NATURAL YOGHURT				
full-fat	6	120	++	++
Greek	8	100	++	++
skimmed-milk	6	50	++	++

Desserts

Definitely excluded!

Desserts can be reintroduced during the weight-maintenance phase, although if you follow the diet you will find your eating patterns are reprogrammed and you no longer desire high-sugar-content foods. All statistics are per 100 grams. The following are examples only; *all* desserts are excluded from a low-carbohydrate diet during the weight-loss phase of the diet.

Food Item	Carbohydrate (g)	Calories	Protein content	Nutritional value
Apple pie	30	200	++	++
Banana split with ice cream	50	300	++	++
Chocolate mousse	30	225	+	+
Chocolate cream	70	45	+	+
Lemon mousse	20	185	+	+
(light)	20	140	+	+
Chocolate sponge pudding	40	210	+	+
Chocolate sundae	25	277	+	+
Christmas pudding	60	340	++	++
Cream lemon desserts	30	285	+	+
Creamed rice	17	100	+	++
Crème caramel	20	120	+	+
CUSTARD				
pouring	15	90	++	++
powder with full-cream milk	12	100	++	++
tart	30	260	+	+
Ice cream, vanilla	24	190	+	+

Food Item	Carbohydrate (g)	Calories	Protein content	Nutritional value
Lemon meringue pie	40	320	+	++
Plum pudding	50	280	++	++
Raspberry mousse	30	245	+	+
Strawberry and cream sundae	17	236	+	+
Strawberry cream trifle	22	170	+	+
Strawberry trifle	18	150	+	+
Trifle	30	100	+	++

Drinks

Drinks vary, so you have to consult the tables. In general terms, tea/decaffeinated coffee/water/diet soft drinks/red and white wine (not sweet)/spirits (in moderation) are *included* and coffee/fruit juices/carbonated soft drinks/beer/cider/sweet wines/milk drinks (even low-fat) are *excluded*.

Drinks included

Food Item	Carbohydrate (g)	Calories	Protein content	Nutritional value
*Coffee (200 ml; decaf)	<1	0	0	0
*DIET SOFT DRINKS (100ml)				
*cola	<1	1	0	0
*lemonade	<1	3	0	0
*orange	<1	1	0	0
*Orangina Light	1	6	<1	0
*tonic	<1	1	0	0
*FRUIT SHOOT (100ml)				
*Orange and peach	<1	5	<1	++
*Light low-sugar orange juice	1	8	tr	++
*SPIRITS (25ml)				
*Bacardi	<1	53	0	0
*bourbon	<1	53	0	0
*brandy	<1	53	0	0
*gin	<1	53	0	0
*rum	<1	53	0	0
*vodka	<1	53	0	0

Food Item	Carbohydrate (g)	Calories	Protein content	Nutritional value
*whisky	<1	53	0	0
*WINE (100ml)				
*red	<1	71	0	0
*white, dry	<1	75	0	0
*white, medium	3	77	0	0
*Sherry (50ml), dry	2	115	0	0
*TEA				
*China	<1	0	0	0
*Sri Lanka	<1	0	0	0
*Vermouth (50ml), dry	2	53	0	0
*WATER				
*carbonated	0	0	0	+++
*flavoured (orange and mango)	0	<1	0	+++
*still	0	0	0	+++

Drinks included – in moderation

Food Item	Carbohydrate (g)	Calories	Protein content	Nutritional value
Certain 'sports' drinks				
Lemon Lucozade Sport	6	28	+	++

Drinks excluded

Food Item	Carbohydrate (g)	Calories	Protein content	Nutritional value
BEER (pint)				
ale	**16–30**	165–320	0	0
bitter	**14**	190	0	0
stout	**10**	200	0	0
CARBONATED SOFT DRINKS (150ml)				
cola	**16**	60	0	0
lemonade	**16**	62	0	0
lemon and lime	**16**	62	0	0
COFFEE, CAFFEINATED (200ml)				
black	**<1**	<1	0	0
cappuccino	**10**	134	++	+
Skinnychino	**10**	70	++	+
white	**3**	25	+	+
CIDER (pint)				
dry	**15**	205	0	0
sweet	**25**	240	0	0
FRUIT JUICE (100ml)				
grapefruit (unsweetened)	**8**	35	0	++
lemon and lime crush	**12**	53	0	++
'Traditional'-style lemonade	**18**	74	0	0
orange, fresh	**8**	33	0	++
commercial (unsweetened)	**9**	37	0	++
MILKSHAKES, THICK (per 100ml)				
chocolate	**20**	120	++	++
strawberry	**20**	120	++	++

Food Item	Carbohydrate (g)	Calories	Protein content	Nutritional value
Port (50ml)	6	75	0	0
SHERRY (50ml)				
medium	3	60	0	0
sweet	4	70	0	0
WINE (100ml)				
rosé	3	75	0	0
white, sweet	6	99	0	0

Eggs

Definitely included!

All statistics are for large hen's eggs unless specified. You can prepare eggs to your preference without increasing the carbohydrate content.

Food Item	Carbohydrate (g)	Calories	Protein content	Nutritional value
*Boiled egg	0	147	++	+++
*Duck's egg (large)	0	160	++	+++
*Fried egg	0	147	++	+++
*Omelette	0	147	++	+++
*Poached egg	0	147	++	+++
*Scrambled egg	0	147	++	+++
*Quail's egg	0	15	++	+++

Fast Food

Definitely excluded!

Fast food essentially means high carbohydrate and high fats which, in turn, mean weight gain. There are a few fast foods (like shish kebabs without the bread) which are essentially low carbohydrate and high protein – but not many! Fast takeaway foods vary tremendously between different manufacturers, so these figures are averages only – but are all too high for an effective diet.

Food Item	Carbohydrate (g)	Calories	Protein content	Nutritional value
Bacon and egg muffin (100g)	25	250	++	++
(per muffin)	33	380	++	++
Big Mac	44	490	+++	++
Cheeseburger (100g)	30	250	++	++
(per burger)	33	300	++	++
Chicken dippers (100g)	13	280	++	++
(per dipper)	2	50	++	++
Chicken, fried (100g)	25	230	++	++
(per piece, approx)	45	420	++	++
Chicken McNuggets (per 6)	12	250	++	++
(per nugget)	2	42	++	++
Chicken nuggets (100g)	15	125	++	++
(per nugget)	3	24	++	++
CHIPS				
fried (100g)	30	190	+	+
oven (100g)	30	160	+	+
takeaway (100g)	30	240	+	+

Food Item	Carbohydrate (g)	Calories	Protein content	Nutritional value
FRENCH FRIES				
oven-bake (100g)	36	240	+	+
(per portion)	28	220	+	+
takeaway (100g)	34	280	+	+
Hamburger, takeaway				
(per burger)	33	250	++	++
Hash brown (100g)	30	230	+	+
(per piece)	15	120	+	+
McChicken Sandwich				
(per sandwich)	38	375	+++	+++
Onion bhaji (100g)	16	300	+	+
(per bhaji)	4	65	+	+
PIZZA (all varieties excluded)				
average pizza (100g)	33	250	+	+
(per slice)	25	170	+	+
cheese and tomato, deep				
pan (100g)	45	310	++	+
(per slice)	45	310	++	+
cheese and tomato, thin				
and crispy (100g)	28	260	++	+
(per slice)	25	230	++	+
four cheese, thin and				
crispy (100g)	32	250	++	+
(per slice)	20	155	++	+
pepperoni (100g)	32	267	++	+
(per slice)	20	164	++	+
vegetable and goat's				
cheese, thin and				
crispy (100g)	31	250	++	+
(per slice)	21	165	++	+

Food Item	Carbohydrate (g)	Calories	Protein content	Nutritional value
Quarter Pounder (100g)	20	240	++	++
(per burger)	37	420	++	++
Saffron rice (100g)	24	155	+	+
Sausage roll (100g)	25	300	+	+
(per roll)	30	370	+	+
Shepherd's pie, beef (100g)	10	95	+	+
(per small pie)	18	180	+	+
Shepherd's pie, lamb (100g)	11	100	+	+
(per small pie)	24	220	+	+
Spring roll (100g)	25	230	+	+
(per roll)	50	400	+	+
Vegetable pakora (100g)	20	265	+	+
(per pakora)	5	60	+	+
Vegetable samosa (100g)	25	225	+	+
(per samosa)	7	60	+	+

Fish and Shellfish

Definitely included!

Fish and shellfish are included *virtually without restriction.*

All figures are for 100 grams of seafood, unless otherwise stated.

Food Item	Carbohydrate (g)	Calories	Protein content	Nutritional value
Fish				
*Anchovies (25g)	<1	45	++++	++++
*Bass	<1	90	++++	++++
*Bream	<1	135	++++	++++
*Calamari	<1	70	++++	++++
*Caviar (20g)	<1	50	++++	++++
*COD	<1	80	++++	++++
breaded fillet (100g)	15	200	+++	+++
(per fillet)	20	250	+++	+++
*Dover sole	<1	80	++++	++++
*Flounder	<1	70	++++	++++
*HADDOCK				
*fresh	<1	100	++++	++++
*smoked	<1	100	++++	++++
*Herring	<1	230	++++	++++
*Kipper	<1	205	++++	++++
*Lemon sole	<1	95	++++	++++
*MACKEREL				
*peppered	<1	355	+++	++++
*smoked	<1	190	++++	++++

Food Item	Carbohydrate (g)	Calories	Protein content	Nutritional value
*SALMON				
*fresh	<1	200	++++	++++
*tinned	<1	150	++++	++++
*smoked	<1	180	++++	++++
*SARDINES				
*fresh	<1	65	++++	++++
*tinned (in oil)	<1	220	++++	++++
*Swordfish	<1	120	++++	++++
*TROUT				
*rainbow	<1	125	++++	++++
*smoked	<1	135	++++	++++
*TUNA				
*fresh	<1	120	++++	++++
*tinned (oil)	<1	180	++++	++++
*tinned (brine)	<1	105	++++	++++
*Whiting	<1	90	++++	++++
Prepared Fish Products				
*Cod fillets	<1	76	+++	+++
Fish fingers (100g)	13	170	++	++
(each)	4	50	++	++
*Haddock fillets	<1	73	+++	+++
Shellfish				
*Clams	<1	80	++++	++++
*Cockles	<1	50	++++	++++
*CRAB				
*fresh	<1	120	++++	++++
*tinned	1	80	++++	++++
*Lobster	<1	120	++++	++++
*Mussels	<1	88	++++	++++
*Oysters	<1	120	++++	++++

Food Item	Carbohydrate (g)	Calories	Protein content	Nutritional value
*Prawns	<1	100	++++	++++
*Scallops	<1	100	++++	++++
*Whelks	<1	50	++++	++++
Prepared shellfish products				
Prawn cocktail	5	188	+++	+++

Fruit

Definitely restricted!

No more than 15 grams of carbohydrate from this source per day, which is approximately a large apple or orange, or 100 grams of blueberries. *Definitely no bananas* which have a very high carbohydrate content. Fruit is very nutritious, and should be reintroduced to your diet after the weight-loss phase is completed.

The statistics quoted are for a single fresh fruit, or the quantity stated. All fruit in syrup is definitely excluded.

Food Item	Carbohydrate (g)	Calories	Protein content	Nutritional value
Apple	10	40	+	+++
Apricot	7	9	+	+++
*Avocado	2	190	+	+++
Banana	31	125	+	++
Blackberries (100g)	12	50	+	+++
Blueberries (100g)	13	52	+	+++
Cherries (100g)	12	52	+	+++
Gooseberries (100g)	13	54	+	+++
Grapefruit	10	51	+	+++
GRAPES (100g)				
black	15	62	+	+++
green	12	55	+	+++
Kiwi fruit	7	35	+	+++
*Lemon	3	11	+	+++
*Lime	<1	8	+	+++
Mandarin	4	20	+	+++

Food Item	Carbohydrate (g)	Calories	Protein content	Nutritional value
Mango	20	80	+	+++
MELON				
honeydew (100g)	6	30	+	+++
rock (100g)	5	22	+	+++
water (100g)	5	22	+	+++
Nectarine	7	32	+	+++
Orange	10	42	+	+++
Passion fruit	3	20	+	+++
Peach	8	33	+	+++
Pear	16	64	+	+++
Pineapple (100g)	8	37	+	+++
Plum	8	34	+	+++
Raspberries (100g)	5	24	+	+++
Rhubarb (100g)	1	8	+	+++
Strawberries (100g)	6	28	+	+++
Tangerine	7	33	+	+++

Herbs and Spices

Definitely included!

Food Item	Carbohydrate (g)	Calories	Protein content	Nutritional value
Fresh herbs (1 tbsp)				
*Basil	<1	15–20	+	+++
*Borage	<1	15–20	+	+++
*Chervil	<1	15–20	+	+++
*Chives	<1	15–20	+	+++
*Coriander	<1	15–20	+	+++
*Dill	<1	15–20	+	+++
*Garlic (1 clove)	<1	3	+	++++
*Horseradish	<1	15–20	+	+++
*Juniper	<1	15–20	+	+++
*Lemon grass	<1	15–20	+	+++
*Marjoram	<1	15–20	+	+++
*Mint	<1	15–20	+	+++
*Oregano	<1	15–20	+	+++
*Parsley	<1	15–20	+	+++
*Rocket (100g)	2	15	+	+++
*Rosemary	<1	15–20	+	+++
*Sage	<1	15–20	+	+++
*Tarragon	<1	15–20	+	+++
*Thyme	<1	15–20	+	+++
*Watercress	2	15–20	+	+++
Dried spices (1 tsp)				
*Allspice	<1	10	tr	++
*Anise	<1	10	tr	++
*Annatto	<1	10	tr	++

Food Item	Carbohydrate (g)	Calories	Protein content	Nutritional value
*Asafoetida	<1	10	tr	++
*Bay leaf	<1	10	tr	++
*Capers	<1	3	tr	++
*Caraway	<1	10	tr	++
*Cassia	<1	10	tr	++
*Chilli powder	<1	10	tr	+++
*Cinnamon	<1	10	tr	++
*Cloves	<1	10	tr	++
*Cumin	<1	10	tr	++
*Curry leaves	<1	10	tr	++
*Fennel	<1	10	tr	++
*Fenugreek	<1	10	tr	++
*Galangal	<1	10	tr	++
*Ginger	7	40	+	+++
*Mustard	<1	10	tr	++
*Nigella	<1	10	tr	++
*Nutmeg	<1	10	tr	++
*Paprika	<1	10	tr	++++
*Pepper	<1	10	tr	++
*Saffron	<1	10	tr	++
*Salt	<1	10	tr	+++
*Sesame	<1	10	tr	+++
*Star anise	<1	10	tr	++
*Szechuan pepper	<1	10	tr	++
*Tamarind	<1	10	tr	++
*Turmeric	<1	10	tr	++
*Vanilla	<1	10	tr	++

Meat

Definitely included!

Meat is included virtually without restriction if 'pure', however there are restrictions on takeaway or prepared varieties.

Food Item	Carbohydrate (g)	Calories	Protein content	Nutritional value
Beef				
*Beefburgers				
*homemade (100g)	0	180	++++	++++
takeaway (100g)	20	250	++	++
*Casserole steak	0	250	++++	++++
*Fillet steak (100g)				
*trimmed	0	190	++++	++++
*untrimmed	0	210	++++	++++
*Heart (100g)	0	180	++++	++++
*Kidney (100g)	0	150	++++	++++
*Liver (100g)	0	200	++++	++++
*Mince, lean (100g)	0	124	++++	++++
*Oxtail (100g)	0	240	++++	++++
*Round steak (100g)				
*trimmed	0	180	++++	++++
*untrimmed	0	200	++++	++++
*Rump steak (100g)				
*trimmed	0	190	++++	++++
*untrimmed	0	270	++++	++++
*Silverside (100g)				
*trimmed	0	160	++++	++++
*untrimmed	0	220	++++	++++

Food Item	Carbohydrate (g)	Calories	Protein content	Nutritional value
*SIRLOIN STEAK (100g)				
*trimmed	0	170	++++	++++
*untrimmed	0	270	++++	++++
*T-BONE STEAK (100g)				
*trimmed	0	140	++++	++++
*untrimmed	0	170	++++	++++
*TOPSIDE STEAK (100g)				
*trimmed	0	150	++++	++++
*untrimmed	0	170	++++	++++
Lamb, natural				
*CHUMP CHOP (70g)				
*trimmed	0	140	++++	++++
*untrimmed	0	200	++++	++++
*CUTLET (40g)				
*trimmed	0	90	++++	++++
*untrimmed	0	130	++++	++++
*Kidney	0	210	++++	++++
*LEG (100g)				
*trimmed	0	200	++++	++++
*untrimmed	0	220	++++	++++
*Liver (100g)	4	230	++++	++++
*LOIN CHOP (50g)				
*trimmed	0	85	++++	++++
*untrimmed	0	180	++++	++++
*SHANK (100g)				
*trimmed	0	140	++++	++++
*untrimmed	0	220	++++	++++
*SHOULDER (100g)				
*trimmed	0	140	++++	++++
*untrimmed	0	260	++++	++++

Food Item	Carbohydrate (g)	Calories	Protein content	Nutritional value
Lamb, commercial				
Lamb and rosemary casserole (100g)	**6**	90	+++	+++
Pork, natural				
*Bacon (100g)	**0**	260	+++	+++
*Fillet (100g)	**0**	170	+++	+++
*LEG (100g)				
*trimmed	**0**	170	+++	+++
*untrimmed	**0**	330	+++	+++
*LOIN CHOP (100g)				
*trimmed	**0**	170	+++	+++
*untrimmed	**0**	350	+++	+++
*MEDALLION (100g)				
*trimmed	**0**	190	+++	+++
*untrimmed	**0**	300	+++	+++
*Mince, lean (100g)	**0**	80	+++	+++
*Spare ribs (100g)	**0**	110	+++	+++
*STEAK (100g)				
*trimmed	**0**	160	+++	+++
*untrimmed	**0**	260	+++	+++
Pork, prepared				
*Gammon steak (100g)	**0**	160	+++	+++
*HAM (100g)				
*trimmed	**0**	100	++++	++++
*untrimmed	**0**	140	+++	+++
*wafer thin	**<1**	105	+++	+++
Pork pie (100g)	**27**	430	+	+
Rabbit				
*trimmed (100g)	**0**	160	+++	+++

Food Item	Carbohydrate (g)	Calories	Protein content	Nutritional value
Veal, natural				
*LEG (100g)				
*trimmed	0	110	+++	+++
*untrimmed	0	130	+++	+++
*Liver (100g)	2	190	+++	++++
*LOIN CHOP (100g)				
*trimmed	0	140	+++	+++
*untrimmed	0	160	+++	+++
*SHOULDER STEAK (100g)				
*trimmed	0	140	+++	+++
*untrimmed	0	150	+++	+++
Veal, prepared				
Schnitzel (100g)	10	330	++	++
Venison				
*Roast venison (100g)	0	200	+++	+++

Nuts

Included in moderation!

Carbohydrate contents of nuts vary so consult the tables. No more than 100g per day, and no more than 50g of *cashew nuts and chestnuts*. The statistics are relevant for 100-gram quantities of raw nuts in each case.

Food Item	Carbohydrate (g)	Calories	Protein content	Nutritional value
Almond	7	610	++	+++
Brazil	3	680	++	+++
Cashew	18	570	++	+++
Chestnut	36	170	+	+++
Hazelnut	6	650	++	+++
Macadamia	5	740	+	+++
Peanut	12	560	++	+++
Pecan	6	690	+	+++
Pine nut	4	690	+++	+++
Pistachio	8	600	++	+++
Walnut	3	690	++	+++

Oils, Mayonnaise and Dressings

Definitely included!

All statistics are based on 100ml. All pure oils are carbohydrate-free, but some oils are much healthier than others. For example, the healthiest oil is undoubtedly extra-virgin olive oil. Olive oil which is not 'virgin' olive oil has most of the nutritional value refined away. Pure mayonnaise is virtually carbohydrate-free, but read the labels on commercial mayonnaise. Some are carbohydrate-free, but some have added sugar – especially those advertised as 'fat-free'. Remember, the calorie content *is irrelevant,* only the carbohydrate content is important in this diet.

Basically vinaigrettes are included in the diet without restriction, however you must *read the label*. Many commercial vinaigrettes have added sugar, and are obviously excluded. Don't bother about the fat content or the calories – just the amount of carbohydrate. The estimates for commercial dressings are variable, depending on the manufacturer, and are intended as a general indication only.

Food Item	Carbohydrate (g)	Calories	Protein content	Nutritional value
Oils				
*Corn oil	0	829	0	+
*Extra-virgin olive oil	0	823	0	++++
*Virgin olive oil	0	822	0	+++
*Olive oil	0	822	0	+
*Grapeseed oil	0	829	0	+

Food Item	Carbohydrate (g)	Calories	Protein content	Nutritional value
*Groundnut oil	0	829	0	++
*Palm oil	0	899	0	+
*Peanut oil	0	899	0	+
*Safflower oil	0	828	0	+
*Sesame oil	0	821	0	++
*Soya oil	0	899	0	+
*Sunflower oil	0	828	0	+
*Wheatgerm oil	0	899	0	++
Mayonnaise and Vinaigrettes				
*Mayonnaise	1	722	+	+
*Vinaigrette, home-made	<1	60	0	++
COMMERCIAL DRESSINGS				
French	15	297	+	+
*low-fat French	9	39	+	+
*Italian	6	120	+	+
*low-fat Italian	7	32	+	+
Thousand Island	20	365	+	+
Teriyaki-style	16	439	+	+
Vinegar (per 15ml)				
*Balsamic	3	10	0	+
*Cider	<1	2	0	+
*Red wine	2	5	0	+
*Rice	<1	5	+	+
*White wine	0	5	0	+

Pasta and Noodles

Definitely excluded!

Pasta and noodles are virtually pure carbohydrate, and must be avoided in the weight-loss phase. The carbohydrate content of commercial products varies, however noodles are basically carbohydrates. All noodles must be excluded during the weight-loss phase of the diet: Chinese, Ho Fen, Hokkien, Mien, Milk Udon, Nama Udon, Ramen, Rice, Rice vermicelli, Shinsu soba, Soba, Somen, Wheatflour, Won ton and Yang chue.

With commercial pasta products, significant variations occur and statistics given are approximations only.

Food Item	Carbohydrate (g)	Calories	Protein content	Nutritional value
Pasta (100g dry weight)				
Acini di pepe	73	360	++	+
Alfabeto	73	360	++	+
Bucatini	73	360	++	+
Cannelloni	73	360	++	+
Cappellettini	73	360	++	+
Casareccia	73	360	++	+
Cavatappi	73	360	++	+
Conchiglie rigate	73	360	++	+
Conchigliette piccole	73	360	++	+
Conchiglioni rigati	73	360	++	+
Corallini	73	360	++	+
Ditali	73	360	++	+
Elicoidali	73	360	++	+
Farfalle	73	360	++	+

Food Item	Carbohydrate (g)	Calories	Protein content	Nutritional value
Farfalloni	73	360	++	+
Farfalloni	73	360	++	+
Fettuccine	73	360	++	+
Fettucelle	73	360	++	+
Fidilini	73	360	++	+
Fricelli	73	360	++	+
Fusilli	73	360	++	+
Fusilli bucati lunghi	73	360	++	+
Gnocchetti sardi	73	360	++	+
Gnocchi	73	360	++	+
Lasagne	73	360	++	+
Lasagnette	73	360	++	+
Linguine	73	360	++	+
Maccheroni	73	360	++	+
Mezze penne rigate	73	360	++	+
Millerighe	73	360	++	+
Orecchiette	73	360	++	+
Orecchiotte	73	360	++	+
Pappardelle	73	360	++	+
Pasta mista	73	360	++	+
Penne lisce	73	360	++	+
Penne rigate	73	360	++	+
Penne mezzane	73	360	++	+
Pennoni	73	360	++	+
Pennoni rigati	73	360	++	+
Perciatelli	73	360	++	+
Pipe rigate	73	360	++	+
Rigatoni	73	360	++	+
Rissoni	73	360	++	+
Rotellini	73	360	++	+

Food Item	Carbohydrate (g)	Calories	Protein content	Nutritional value
Spaccatella	73	360	++	+
Spaghetti	73	360	++	+
Spaghettini	73	360	++	+
Stelline	73	360	++	+
Tagliatelle	73	360	++	+
Tagliarini	73	360	++	+
Tagliolini	73	360	++	+
Tonnarelli	73	360	++	+
Vermicelli	73	360	++	+
Ziti	73	360	++	+
Noodles (100g)				
Egg noodles	70	340	++	+
Commercial pasta products (100g)				
Macaroni cheese	15	120	+	+
Ravioli in tomato sauce	13	73	+	+
Spaghetti hoops	12	56	+	+
Spaghetti in tomato sauce:	13	61	+	+

Poultry

Definitely included!

Poultry is *included virtually without restriction* if 'pure'; however, there are restrictions on takeaway or prepared varieties.

Food Item	Carbohydrate (g)	Calories	Protein content	Nutritional value
Chicken, natural (100g)				
*BREAST				
*skinless	0	170	++++	++++
*with skin	0	210	+++	+++
*DRUMSTICK				
*skinless	0	90	+++	+++
*with skin	0	110	+++	+++
*THIGH				
*skinless	0	60	+++	+++
*with skin	0	70	+++	+++
*WING				
*skinless	0	70	+++	+++
*with skin	0	90	+++	+++
Chicken, prepared (100g)				
*Breast roll	0	120	++++	++++
*Drumsticks	0	180	++++	++++
*Red Thai-style	3	135	+++	+++
*Tikka-style dippers	5	193	+++	+++
*Wings, in barbecue marinade	3	232	+++	+++

Food Item	Carbohydrate (g)	Calories	Protein content	Nutritional value
Duck (100g)				
*ROAST DUCK				
*skinless	0	180	++++	++++
*with skin	0	300	+++	+++
Game (100g)				
*Grouse	0	170	++++	++++
*Partridge	0	210	+++	+++
*Pheasant	0	130	+++	+++
*Pigeon breast	0	200	+++	+++
*Quail, roast	0	130	+++	+++
Turkey, natural (100g)				
*BREAST				
*skinless	0	105	++++	++++
*with skin	0	140	+++	+++
*Mince	0	176	++++	++++
Turkey, prepared (100g)				
*Breast roll	4	92	+++	+++

Pulses

Definitely excluded!

Pulses are nutritionally excellent, but unfortunately have a high natural carbohydrate content. They can – and should – be included in any healthy diet (in moderation), but only after the weight-loss phase has been completed. In the period of active weight loss, pulses are *essentially excluded*. Once again, all statistics relate to 100-gram portions to enable comparisons.

Food Item	Carbohydrate (g)	Calories	Protein content	Nutritional value
Beans				
Aduki	20	120	+++	+++
Baked beans in tomato sauce	14	75	++	++
Black-eye	20	110	+++	+++
Broad	6	150	+++	+++
Butter	12	80	+++	+++
Chickpeas	15	110	+++	+++
Chilli	12	70	+	++
Haricot	16	100	++	++
Hummus	12	190	+++	+++
Kidney (red)	16	100	+++	+++
Lentils	16	100	+++	+++
Lima	10	75	+++	+++
Pinto	25	140	+++	+++
SOYA				
bean	5	140	+++	+++
tofu	1	75	+++	+++

Rice

Definitely excluded!

Although some forms of rice have a much higher nutritional content (for example, wholegrain rice) than others (such as white rice), *all* rice has a very high carbohydrate content, and is *excluded* from the diet. All of the following are excluded: brown rice (long- and short-grain), white rice (long- and short-grain), basmati rice, jasmine rice, glutinous rice, arborio rice, wholegrain rice, carnaroli, sushi Japanese rice, calasparra, Thai (black and white) rice and vialone nano. In other words, *all forms of rice are excluded during the weight loss phase of the diet,* but obviously rice can be included (in moderation) after the active weight-loss phase is over. All statistics refer to 100-gram quantities (dry weight).

Food Item	Carbohydrate (g)	Calories	Protein content	Nutritional value
Arborio	78	350	++	++
Basmati	76	350	++	++
Brown	74	349	++	++
Thai fragrant	77	350	++	++
WHITE RICE				
long-grain	76	340	++	++
short-grain	78	375	++	++
Wholegrain	75	350	++	+++

Sauces, Mustards and Stocks

Included in moderation!

These are *generally included*, but carbohydrate contents vary, so consult the tables. All statistics refer to 100ml, but as the average serving is $1/10$ of this amount, it is usually quite safe to include most sauces in the diet – in moderation! However, only tomato sauce (with the powerful antioxidant lycopene) has a rich nutritional component. Commercial mustards, in particular, vary in carbohydrate contents; the table below provides a general guide, but you must check the individual label.

Food Item	Carbohydrate (g)	Calories	Protein content	Nutritional value
Sauces				
Barbecue	**65**	270	+	+
Chilli	**50**	50	+	+
Chutney	**55**	200	+	+
GRAVY				
commercial	**10**	130	+	+
powder	**5**	25	+	+
Hoisin	**38**	180	+	+
Horseradish	**10**	105	+	
HP	**27**	119	+	+
Mango chutney	**58**	230	+	+
Mint, no added sugar	**0**	0	+	+++
Oyster	**35**	190	+	+
PASTA SAUCES, COMMERCIAL				
Bolognese	**9**	52	+	++
Chargrilled vegetable	**9**	60	+	+++
Pesto	**60**	550	+	++

Food Item	Carbohydrate (g)	Calories	Protein content	Nutritional value
Salsa, fresh	8	47	+	++
Satay	35	450	+	+
Seafood	20	335	+	+
Soy	8	40	+	+
Sweet and sour	25	100	+	+
Tartare	14	263	+	+
Tomato	35	155	+	+++
Tomato ketchup	25	107	+	+++
White sauce, homemade	20	200	++	++
Worcestershire	25	110	+	+
Mustard				
English	19	190	++	++
French	4	104	++	++
Wholegrain	4	140	++	++
Commercial stocks				
BISTO				
chicken gravy granules	56	389	+	+
original	55	390	+	+
vegetarian granules	55	394	+	+
KNORR STOCK CUBES				
beef	21	326	++	++
chicken	24	301	++	++
lamb	16	295	++	++
vegetable	22	308	++	++
OXO STOCK CUBES				
beef	38	265	++	++
chicken	37	243	++	++
lamb	43	289	++	++
vegetable	42	253	++	++

Soups

Read the label! The carbohydrate content of tinned and packaged soups varies tremendously between manufacturers; some have a relatively high carbohydrate content, others a much lower one. Commercial soups with a lower carbohydrate content are included here. An average serving of 200ml can be safely included in a low-carbohydrate diet.

Obviously the homemade variety can be safely included in the diet – providing it follows a low-carbohydrate recipe. Homemade soups vary tremendously in carbohydrate and nutritional content, and therefore I would refer you to *The New High Protein Diet Cookbook* for a selection of highly nutritious, low-carbohydrate homemade soup recipes.

Food Item	Carbohydrate (g)	Calories	Protein content	Nutritional value
Commercial soups				
Autumn vegetable (100ml)	8	40	+	++
(per serving)	16	80	+	++
Chicken noodle (100ml)	5	27	+	++
(per serving)	10	54	+	++
Cream of chicken (100ml)	5	51	+	++
(per serving)	10	102	+	++
Cream of tomato (100ml)	11	71	+	++
(per serving)	22	142	+	++
Cream of mushroom (100ml)	5	51	+	++
(per serving)	10	102	+	++
French onion (100ml)	5	25	+	++
(per serving)	10	50	+	++

Food Item	Carbohydrate (g)	Calories	Protein content	Nutritional value
Lentil (100ml)	8	41	+	++
(per serving)	16	82	+	++
Minestrone (100ml)	5	30	+	++
(per serving)	10	60	+	++
Mulligatawny (100ml)	7	60	+	++
(per serving)	14	120	+	++
Pea and ham (100ml)	9	51	++	++
(per serving)	18	102	++	++
Scotch broth (100ml)	7	46	+	++
(per serving)	14	92	+	++
Spicy tomato and rice (100ml)	9	45	+	++
(per serving)	18	90	+	++
Vegetable (100ml)	8	47	+	++
(per serving)	16	94	+	++

Vegetables and Vegetable Products

Definitely included!

Apart from those with a high carbohydrate content, such as potatoes or parsnips, vegetables are included virtually without restriction on this diet. Obviously, vegetables have many different shapes and sizes; for standardization (and to allow you to compare like with like), all statistics refer to 100 grams of each fresh vegetable.

Food Item	Carbohydrate (g)	Calories	Protein content	Nutritional value
Low-carbohydrate vegetables				
*Alfalfa sprouts	4	30	+	+++
*ARTICHOKE				
*globe	1	8	++	+++
Jerusalem	9	40	++	+++
*Asparagus	1	12	+	+++
*Aubergine	2	14	+	+++
*BEANS				
*French	4	25	+	+++
*green	4	25	+	+++
Beetroot	8	35	+	+++
*Broccoli	1	25	++	+++
*Brussels sprouts	2	25	++	+++
*CABBAGE				
*bok choy	<1	12	+	+++
*Chinese	<1	8	+	+++
*red	2	22	+	+++

Food Item	Carbohydrate (g)	Calories	Protein content	Nutritional value
*savoy	2	20	+	+++
Carrots	8	37	+	+++
*Cauliflower	2	20	+	+++
*Celeriac	5	30	+	+++
*Celery	3	12	+	+++
*CHILLI				
*green	1	20	+	+++
*red	4	26	+	+++
*COURGETTES				
*green	2	15	+	+++
*yellow	2	15	+	+++
*CUCUMBER				
English	6	9	+	+++
*Lebanese	3	12	+	+++
*Fennel	4	12	+	+++
*Herb salad, commercial	2	15	+	+++
*Kale	2	33	++	++++
*LEEK				
*standard	3	20	+	+++
*baby	3	23	+	+++
*LETTUCE				
*cos	2	20	+	+++
*curly endive	2	20	+	+++
*green lollo	2	20	+	+++
*green oak	2	20	+	+++
*iceberg	2	20	+	+++
*lollo rosso	2	20	+	+++
*mesclun	2	20	+	+++
*radicchio	2	20	+	+++
*red oak	2	20	+	+++
*Swiss chard	2	20	+	+++

Food Item	Carbohydrate (g)	Calories	Protein content	Nutritional value
*Mangetout	5	60	++	+++
*Marrow	4	20	+	+++
*MUSHROOMS				
*button	2	25	+	+++
Chinese	15	50	+	+++
enoki	6	35	+	+++
oyster	5	35	+	+++
*ONION				
*brown	4	25	+	++++
*red	4	25	+	++++
*white	4	25	+	++++
*PEAS				
fresh green	6	60	+	+++
tinned	9	67	+	+
sugarsnap	5	33	+	+++
*PEPPERS				
*green	3	15	+	++++
*red	4	25	+	++++
Pumpkin	7	40	+	+++
*Radish	2	3	+	+++
*Salad leaves, commercial	2	25	+	+++
*Seaweed	<1	10	+	+++
*Shallot	4	25	+	++++
*Spinach	2	30	+	+++
*Spring onion	4	25	+	++++
*Swede	2	10	+	+++
*TOMATO				
*beefsteak	3	20	+	++++
*cherry	3	20	+	++++
*plum	3	20	+	++++
*plum, tinned/peeled	4	24	+	++++

Food Item	Carbohydrate (g)	Calories	Protein content	Nutritional value
purée	18	92	++	++++
*round	3	20	+	++++
*vine-ripened	3	20	+	++++
*Turnip	2	12	++	+++

High-carbohydrate vegetables

Food Item	Carbohydrate (g)	Calories	Protein content	Nutritional value
Cassava	30	125	+	+++
Mushrooms, shiitake, dried	64	295	++	+++
Parsnip	14	65	+	+++
Potato	16	75	+	+++
Sweet potato	20	80	+	+++
Tomato, sun-dried, in oil	25	200	+	+++
Yam	35	150	+	+++

Commercially prepared vegetables

Food Item	Carbohydrate (g)	Calories	Protein content	Nutritional value
Mushroom provençale: (mushrooms, tomatoes, onions, garlic and herbs)	4	50	+	+++
SAUSAGES, VEGETARIAN organic leek and cheese (100g)	11	195	++	++
(per sausage)	5	81	++	++
Vegetable selection: (potatoes, broccoli, carrots and spring greens)	6	80	+	+++
Vegetarian quarter pounder burgers	7	164	+++	+++

Essential Nutrition for Health

Nutrition is, quite simply, the 'goodness' in our food. The essential nutrients in food keep us healthy, and an excess of non-essential foods (which, by definition, are unnecessary) will ultimately be harmful to health. And nutrition is a very simple concept to understand, it has merely been made somewhat incomprehensible by some 'experts' in the field. The essential nutrients, without which we cannot survive, are:

- proteins
- certain essential fats
- vitamins
- minerals.

The most obvious omission from the above list is carbohydrates. In other words, *carbohydrates are not essential, or even necessary, for health.* Carbohydrates provide energy, nothing else, and energy can be obtained from proteins and fats. Foods containing natural *unrefined* carbohydrates (such as those in vegetables and fruits) also contain many other essential vitamins and minerals, and are therefore healthy. However, *refined* carbohydrates (such as those in biscuits, cakes, confectionery, white bread, white pasta and white rice) contain virtually no nutrition, and should therefore be restricted.

Protein

Protein is essential in our diet, as it is broken down into its component parts (amino acids), which are then re-formed as our own body proteins. *Complete* proteins are those which contain all of the essential amino acids for health, and are found only in animal products (meat, poultry, fish, shellfish and dairy produce) or soya products. Plant sources are *incomplete* proteins, as they do not contain all of the amino acids we need in order to build our own body proteins. However, all essential amino acids can be obtained by combining grain products (such as rice) with pulses (such as beans).

In essence, it is much easier to obtain all of the essential amino acids for health with a diet that contains meat, fish or poultry, but it is quite possible to obtain all on a properly balanced vegetarian diet.

Essential fatty acids

The simple fact is that we all need certain fats for health. We don't need carbohydrates, but we do need fats. Of course, the fats that we need are not those in chips and pizza. The essential fatty acids are omega-3 and omega-6 fatty acids.

Omega-3 fatty acids are found in so-called 'fatty' fish, such as herring, mackerel, sardines, salmon and tuna. To a lesser extent, they are also present in egg yolks, nuts and seed oils (such as flaxseed).

Omega-6 fatty acids are present in certain seeds and their oils (particularly safflower, sunflower and sesame), egg yolks, wholegrains and certain vegetables.

Other fats, such as those in virgin olive oils, are not *essential* for health, but are certainly very *beneficial* to a healthy lifestyle. And remember, you should always select 'virgin', or preferably 'extra-virgin' olive oils, as these have not been processed; the more the oils are processed, the less nutrition they will contain.

Fats to avoid, or at least reduce to minimal quantities, are those combined with carbohydrates, as in chips, pizza, crisps, cakes, pastries, biscuits, chocolate and confectionery. The carbohydrates in these foods will stimulate insulin production, which will instantly convert the dietary fat to body fat. If you don't eat carbohydrates, the 'pure' fats in omega-3, omega-6 and virgin olive oils will *not* be converted to body fat.

Vitamins

Vitamins are chemicals which we require to facilitate the millions of chemical reactions which take place in every cell of our body every second. Although they are required only in minute quantities, without them we become very sick and may die. Many people have heard of scurvy, caused by a lack of vitamin C, which causes problems with blood clotting. This disease used to be the cause of death for many sailors on long voyages, until it was discovered that citrus fruits (which contain large quantities of vitamin C) completely prevented the condition.

Vitamin deficiency causes many millions of deaths throughout the world. Fortunately, this is not common in the United Kingdom, but lesser degrees of vitamin deficiency can cause serious debility and reduced immunity, leading to increased liability to infections. Probably the most common vitamin deficiency in the United Kingdom is vitamin D deficiency, which causes osteoporosis.

The important fact is that you *must* have a balanced diet to obtain all of the necessary vitamins and minerals for optimum health. This does *not* simply involve having any five portions of fruit and vegetables per day, as this may not provide all of the essential vitamins you require for good health. For example, a typical diet may include fruit such as strawberries, apples, pears, or bananas, and vegetables such as potatoes, mushrooms, iceberg lettuce, cauliflower and chickpeas. All of these fruits and vegetables are very healthy and nutritious, but they all share a common deficiency: *they are all low in vitamin A.* These wonderful foods have many other essential vitamins, but this merely demonstrates that if you blindly follow the 'five portions of fruit and vegetables a day' dogma, you may not be as healthy as you expect. It is absolutely essential to eat a *combination* of foods which will provide *all* of the essential vitamins and minerals for health. And this is actually very easy to achieve. We certainly do not wish to overwhelm you with long lists of vitamin and mineral content in foods. That is a waste of time, and actually counter-productive, as lists of that nature can simply turn you off the subject. Of much more importance is to provide *brief* lists of the main foods containing the essential vitamins and minerals, and to demonstrate how these are easily incorporated into delicious recipes which are practical for modern life; the recipes are included in *The New High Protein Diet* and *The New High Protein Diet Cookbook*.

There are many vitamins which are essential for health. A deficiency of any single one will cause health problems sooner or later, so you can appreciate that it is *absolutely essential* that you incorporate all of the vitamins in a healthy, balanced diet. The main vitamins and their most important sources are as follows:

Vitamin A

Vitamin A is essential for many different chemical reactions in all cells of the body. It has antioxidant properties, which have a major role in maintaining health and preventing ageing. It is also essential for night vision.

This vitamin is present in particularly high concentration in red and yellow vegetables, such as carrots, red peppers and tomatoes; but also in many green leafy vegetables such as kale and spinach. Fruit with a high concentration of this vitamin include mangoes, rock melon and gooseberries. The only animal source of vitamin A in significant quantity is liver, although there are reasonable concentrations in eggs (especially duck eggs), butter, cheeses, cream and salmon. Herbs and spices (such as chilli, coriander, dill, paprika and parsley) contain very high concentrations of this essential antioxidant.

Vitamin B

There is no individual vitamin B, but rather a group of separate vitamins, each essential in its own right:

VITAMIN B1 (THIAMIN)

Thiamin is an essential contributing factor in many of the chemical reactions involved in the release of energy from carbohydrates, fats and proteins.

The highest concentrations of vitamin B1 are found in pork, salmon, other meats and fish to a much lesser degree, wholemeal flour and certain other cereals (such as pearl barley); certain nuts (especially brazils, cashews, raw peanuts and pistachios); sunflower seeds, and legumes (such as kidney beans). In general, most fruit and vegetables are a poor source of vitamin B1.

VITAMIN B2 (RIBOFLAVIN)

Vitamin B2 is also essential for the effective release of energy from foods. It is required for the proper functioning of the nervous system, the eyes and the skin.

Riboflavin is added to some foods, principally processed cereals; however, the highest *natural* sources of vitamin B2 are in liver and kidneys, dairy products (milk, cheese and yoghurt), meat, poultry, eggs, fish, shellfish (especially crab), some nuts (particularly almonds and brazil nuts), mushrooms and broad beans. Once again, in general, fruit and vegetables are low in vitamin B2.

VITAMIN B3 (NIACIN)

As with many other vitamins in the B group, vitamin B3 is essential for the chemical conversion of food to energy, which takes place in every cell of the body.

The highest concentrations of vitamin B3 are found in fish (especially tuna and salmon), liver, meat, chicken, wholegrain products, cheese, legumes (especially soya beans), sunflower seeds and peanuts. Fruit and vegetables are, in general, a relatively poor source of vitamin B3.

VITAMIN B6 (PYRIDOXINE)

This vitamin is essential for the conversion of proteins to energy. It is found primarily in wheat germ, wholemeal products, meat (especially pork) and poultry, fish (particularly tuna and salmon), certain nuts (peanuts, hazelnuts, cashews and walnuts), avocados and legumes (especially lentils and soy beans). Dairy products are a poor source of vitamin B6, and most fruits contain little vitamin B6 (with the notable exception of bananas). Similarly, most vegetables contain little vitamin B6, except capsicum, onions, potatoes and tomatoes.

FOLATE

Folate is a member of the B group of vitamins, but was discovered at a time when the allocation of 'numbers' to the group had been discontinued. Once again, this is an essential nutrient in our diet, responsible for many different functions including the manufacture of DNA (our genes) and the production of amino acids (such as methionine), which are the 'building blocks' of structural proteins.

It is present in highest concentrations in liver and kidneys, vegetables (especially beetroot, asparagus, kale and spinach), wholegrain cereals, nuts (such as cashews, peanuts and hazelnuts), legumes, mussels and sunflower seeds. Lower, but significant, quantities are present in cheese and milk, meat, poultry and fish (however, more substantial concentrations are present in tuna and salmon). Many fruits are a good source of folate, especially melons, blackberries, oranges and strawberries.

VITAMIN B12

Vitamin B12 is the only vitamin which is *not* present in foods of plant origin. It acts in conjunction with folate in the production of DNA in all cells of the body, and is essential (with folate) in the development of red blood cells. Lack of vitamin B12 leads to the condition called pernicious anaemia.

Highest concentrations are present in liver, kidneys, oysters, mussels and some fish, especially sardines and salmon. Beef, dairy products, eggs (particularly duck eggs), pork and most other fish are lesser sources of vitamin B12. Nuts, fruit, vegetables and legumes contain none of this essential vitamin.

Vitamin C

Vitamin C is essential for many different functions in every cell in the body. It acts as a 'co-enzyme', allowing enzymes (proteins which facilitate chemical reactions in the cells) to function. It is particularly important in the formation of collagen, and is present in teeth, gums, bones and blood capillaries. It is an essential component in blood clotting and nervous function. Perhaps the most important role of vitamin C is its antioxidant function, preventing free radical formation which is an important factor in the ageing process.

The best dietary sources of vitamin C are fruit (especially blackcurrants, lemons, oranges, mangoes and strawberries) and vegetables, of which the highest concentrations are present in capsicum (red more than green capsicum), broccoli, Brussels sprouts, kale, chilli and parsley. The only significant animal sources of vitamin C are liver and kidneys. Milk contains a minimal amount of vitamin C, and there is effectively none in meat, poultry, fish, eggs, cheese and nuts.

Vitamin D

This vitamin is essential for the body to absorb and use calcium, the levels of which must be carefully controlled to allow nerve and muscle function, especially that of the heart muscle.

Vitamin D is manufactured by our skin in sunlight. However, the highest dietary sources are fatty fish: herring, mackerel, sardines, salmon and, to a lesser extent, tuna. There are much lesser amounts in cream, butter, cheese and eggs, and small amounts in liver. Nuts, avocados, plants, other meats and vegetable oils effectively contain no vitamin D.

Vitamin E

Vitamin E is an antioxidant, preventing the formation of free radicals; it helps to prevent ageing and increases immunity to infection.

There are very few cases of deficiency of this vitamin. It is primarily found in wheat germ products, fatty fish (herring, salmon, sardines and tuna), shellfish (especially prawns and mussels), calamari, certain vegetable oils (sunflower and safflower), nuts (especially almonds, hazelnuts, peanuts and pine nuts) and wholegrain products. White fish are low in vitamin E, and there is very little in meat, dairy products, eggs, most fruit (except avocados and blackberries) and most vegetables, except cabbage, aubergines, mushrooms, sweet potatoes and tomato purée.

Vitamin K

Vitamin K is provided from our diet and is also manufactured by bacteria in the intestine. The primary function of this vitamin is in the manufacture of proteins which are essential for clotting of the blood.

It is present in high concentrations in green vegetables, especially broccoli, Brussels sprouts, kale, lettuce, cabbage, spinach and parsley. Poor sources of vitamin K include meat, poultry, fish, dairy products, eggs, grains and most fruit (with the exception of avocado).

Minerals

Minerals are natural elements which are present in the earth and which are therefore also present in the foods we eat. Like vitamins, they do *not* provide energy, and therefore cannot be converted to fat. Their essential function is to facilitate chemical reactions in every cell of the body, and many minerals are essential for health (in small quantities). Although most of the essential functions of minerals are hidden from view, some are very obvious, like the presence of calcium in teeth and bones.

There are many essential minerals. The following list is not comprehensive, but merely intended to provide an indication of the functions of some of the essential minerals for health and their sources in different food groups.

Calcium

This mineral is essential for many functions of the body, especially the formation of structural proteins (such as teeth and bones), the regulation of heart muscle function, and the regulation of the nervous system.

Calcium is present in a diverse range of foods, however, the highest dietary source is undoubtedly cheese, especially Parmesan. Emmental, Edam, Gruyère and Cheddar also have a high calcium content. Lesser amounts are present in tofu, sardines, salmon, nuts (especially almonds and hazelnuts), green vegetables (such as kale, spinach and watercress) and dairy products.

Chromium

Chromium is particularly important in the regulation of insulin, and therefore essential for the body to regulate fat metabolism. It is very important in the utilization of glucose by the body, and essential in a healthy diet.

This element has a high concentration in eggs, meat, cheese, wine, wholegrain products, apples, potatoes and butter. In general, other fruit and vegetables are a poor source of chromium.

Copper

Copper acts in conjunction with folate in the formation of the nervous system. It is essential for the effective absorption of iron from the intestine, and therefore essential for the prevention of anaemia.

The highest levels of copper are found in liver, shellfish (especially oysters, whelks, winkles, crab and lobster), seeds (sunflower and sesame), tomato purée and nuts (especially cashews and brazil nuts).

Iodine

This element is absolutely essential for the function of the thyroid gland which produces the hormone thyroxine. Lack of this hormone has multiple effects on the body, with slowing of metabolism, slowing of the heart rate, fatigue and weight gain as the main consequences.

Iodine is found primarily in products from the sea, such as marine fish, shellfish and seaweed, although vegetables grown in areas which have an iodine-rich soil are also good sources of this mineral.

Iron

Although iron performs essential functions in every cell of the body, most of the iron is present in the red blood cells, where it is essential for the transport of oxygen to every cell in the body. Lack of iron is the main cause of anaemia.

Iron is found in many different foods. The best sources of this mineral include shellfish (especially cockles and mussels), liver, seeds (such as sesame and sunflower), wheat germ, parsley, nuts (cashews and pine nuts), eggs and meat.

Manganese

Manganese has an essential role in glucose metabolism and in the production of cholesterol and the utilization of body fats. It is also essential for the production of hormones.

The highest concentrations of this mineral are found in wheat germ, nuts (especially pine nuts, hazelnuts and pecan nuts), seeds (sunflower and sesame) and wholemeal products.

Phosphorus

Phosphorus is universally present in the cells of the body, with many essential functions including the effective absorption of vitamins B2 and B3 from the intestine, and the formation of bones. It is particularly important for those on a weight-reducing diet as it plays an important role in the breakdown of body fat.

This essential mineral is present in a wide range of foods, especially wheat germ, seeds (sunflower and sesame), nuts (particularly pine nuts, brazils and cashews), cheese, eggs, liver and poultry.

Potassium

Potassium acts in conjunction with sodium to regulate the transfer of fluid between cells, and is essential for the regulation of the heart and muscle function. It is also essential for the effective metabolism of carbohydrates and proteins.

It is particularly prevalent in dried fruits (such as apricots, raisins and sultanas), nuts (pine nuts, almonds, and peanuts), parsley and coriander, sunflower seeds, garlic, fish and avocados. Lesser amounts are present in milk and in other fruit and vegetables.

Selenium

Selenium has essential functions as an antioxidant, assisting in the removal of free radicals from the body and therefore helping to prevent ageing and resistance to disease. It is also essential in the manufacture of thyroid hormones.

Particularly high sources of this mineral include nuts (especially brazil nuts), sea fish, shellfish (lobster, squid, scallops and prawns) and sunflower seeds. Lesser amounts are present in pork, eggs, poultry and cheese.

Sodium

Sodium is an essential element which acts in combination with potassium to regulate the transfer of fluid across the cell membranes. Even a slight imbalance can cause serious health problems. It is particularly important for effective function of the nervous system and the heart rate.

Sodium is universally present in many diverse foods, including stock cubes, soy sauce, prawns, pork, smoked salmon and tomato ketchup. Lesser amounts are found in cheese, eggs and dairy products.

Sulphur

Sulphur is an integral component of insulin, and is essential for the immune system to combat infections. It is a component of certain amino acids, and is present in many structural proteins, including hair, nails and skin.

This element is present in mustard, poultry, nuts (especially peanuts and brazils), pork, liver, fish (particularly kippers), beef, cheese and eggs. Legumes and certain other vegetables (Brussels sprouts and cabbage) are also good sources of this mineral.

Zinc

Zinc is a factor in many essential body functions. It is a component of insulin (and is therefore essential in the metabolism of carbohydrates), enables effective function of the immune system, and is required for the manufacture of proteins.

The highest concentrations of zinc are present in oysters, wheat germ, liver, shellfish, beef, nuts (pine nuts and cashews), and cheese (Parmesan and Emmental). Lesser amounts are present in eggs, Cheddar cheese, chicken and milk.